"God, What Is Happening to Me?"

"God, What Is Happening to Me?"

❧

Karen Turner

God, What Is Happening to Me?

© 2016 Karen Turner, CHHC, LMT, AADP

For information, contact Karen Turner at LivingWell@myfairpoint.net.

The content of this book is for general informational purposes only.

It is not meant to be used, nor should it be used, to diagnose or treat any medical condition or to replace the services of your physician or other health care provider. The advice and strategies contained in the book may not be suitable for all readers.

Please consult your health care provider for any questions that you may have about your own medical situation. Neither the author, publisher, IIN nor any of their employees or representatives guarantee the accuracy of information in this book or its usefulness to a particular reader, nor are they responsible for any damages or negative consequences that may result from any treatment, action taken, or inaction by any person reading or following the information in this book.

To contact the author, visit KarenLTurner.com.

All scriptures are from the King James Version.

ISBN-13: 9781537662428
ISBN-10: 1537662422
Library of Congress Control Number: 2016917907
CreateSpace Independent Publishing Platform
North Charleston, South Carolina

Printed in the United States of America.

Table of Contents

Introduction

๛

"I CAN'T GO IN THE grocery store! I can't go in! It's too much!" Instead, I sit in my car and cry. After twenty minutes, I put on my sunglasses, take a deep breath, and go in. My heart is pounding as I scan every aisle. If I see someone I know, I push my cart to a different aisle. I can't see anyone I know! They will ask how I am doing, and I will start crying and fall apart. I will be so embarrassed, mostly because I don't know why I am feeling this way. "Keep going," I tell myself, "You're almost done." I make it to the register and hope the checkout girl doesn't talk to me. I'm thinking, "Hurry up, bag my groceries, get me out of here—I want to go home! What is wrong with me? Oh God, I think I'm cracking up!"

Do you experience similar, strange symptoms? Do you cry for no reason? Are you having anxiety about making supper? Do you feel like you are not yourself at times? Are you having heart palpitations? This scene and many others in this book may sound familiar to you. My intention for writing this book is to *share my experiences in the hope that you may recognize some of these symptoms in yourself and be able to put a name to them.* It is a very scary place to be when you are having anxiety about normal, everyday things, feeling like you have cobwebs in your head, and crying often for no apparent reason.

This transition snuck up on me. It didn't all happen in one day—a little here and a little there. The symptoms by themselves didn't mean much, but all together they meant one thing: I was going through *the change*! I couldn't function the same anymore; my feelings and thoughts scared me. I was forty-two when strange things started happening; I thought I was losing my mind—I had no idea what was going on inside of me.

No one really talked about the change. I don't remember my mom ever saying anything to me when I was younger. I did ask her once, and all she said was, "Oh is that when you get hot?" My health care provider didn't warn me, and I certainly don't remember what was taught in my fifth grade health class. I may have seen commercials on TV for hot flashes, but they never mentioned the rest of the symptoms. It's as if they didn't exist. I was also older than most of my friends; they were still having babies, so they couldn't help me. I was on my own with this one.

While speaking with a friend who was about six years older, I confessed to her how I had been feeling. She told me I wasn't losing my mind but that I was going through menopause. "What? Menopause? Are you kidding me?" She told me that when she went through it, her behavior changed, and she would lose patience with her coworkers and even yell at them. I was shocked; as she was a woman I looked up to, the nicest person I knew, and a Bible teacher at that. She encouraged me to read *The Wisdom of Menopause*, by Christiane Northrup, MD. I got a copy of this book and read, read, and read! I was amazed as I saw myself on almost every page of the book. I said to my husband, "Hon, listen to what this book says. It sounds just like me." My condition had a name: *perimenopause*. I was relieved to know I was not going off my rocker!

There are many symptoms—both physical and emotional—as this book will describe. I will admit I didn't want to be in perimenopause, because it meant that I was getting older. Although perimenopause has been portrayed negatively, it can also be a wonderful time. For the first time as an adult, I was able to focus on myself instead of others.

I think it is extremely important that women are prepared for this time of life; it is cruel not to share what is coming. Moms tell their teens about menstruation—why not perimenopause? We, women, must learn how to take care of ourselves during this time of hormonal shifting and upheaval. We must educate ourselves and get support from women who are in it and have been through it. The beginning is a scary time until we figure out what is happening. Since perimenopause can last many years, we must prepare ourselves for unchartered territory. Learn about the symptoms so that when they come, you are ready for them. This will help take the fear out of your journey.

I wrote this book to save at least one woman from the fear of not knowing what is happening to her mind and body. If you are that woman, I want you to know that this physical and emotional process is normal, and you are normal. In the first chapter, you will learn what perimenopause is. Next, you will learn the symptoms. Chapter 3 will teach tips on how to handle the symptoms. Chapter 4 will explain how to eat better, and chapter 5 will give you spiritual encouragement for this journey. Also, I have included journaling pages for you to write down your feelings and kind thoughts about yourself—a process that you will learn more about as you read this book.

There are things you can do to adjust and make your life a little easier as you go through the change. I encourage you to read the rest of this book to identify what may be happening to you both physically and emotionally. Then, take advantage of helpful tips that may help you through this time. I believe this book will help make your transition easier; you will have much less fear and a purse full of tools to assist you.

Ladies, you cannot skip over menopause. The only way out is *through* and you need the support of experienced women for this time of life. I understand what you are going through, and I am giving each of you a big, long, loving, compassionate hug!

CHAPTER 1

Perimenopause

᛭

What Is It?

The prefix "peri" means "around," so it is the time around menopause. Just as it takes time for a girl to transition into being a menstruating teenager and being able to bear children, it takes time for a woman to transition into *not being able* to bear children. With the average age of menopause being fifty-one, perimenopause is the time leading up to the end of this change. A woman is said to be *in menopause* when she has not had a period for one year. This is the result of the gradual changes that occur during perimenopause.

I will not get too technical here. Basically, what occurs is that our estrogen and progesterone hormones fluctuate during perimenopause. These hormones do specific things in our bodies, and they also affect our thinking and emotions. For instance, the physiological effect of excess estrogen decreases sex drive, and progesterone restores sex drive. The effect of estrogen dominance—or imbalance of estrogen because of too little progesterone—is poor sleep patterns, whereas, progesterone promotes normal sleep patterns. The same goes with depression, anxiety, and headaches. Progesterone is an antidepressant and calms anxiety. When these hormones fluctuate (and there is no neat pattern for this), you may have symptoms like PMS or feel "all over the map" emotionally and physically, daily and sometimes hourly.

When Does It Begin and End?

Perimenopause usually begins in your forties, but you may notice some changes in your midthirties. Just as every woman's body is unique, perimenopause will last somewhere from two to fifteen years or more. As I look back, I started noticing symptoms in my early forties.

Perimenopause ends when it ends. I am fifty-seven now and have not had a period for seven years, but I still have some symptoms.

Invisible Inside Work

Except for the first three months, everyone can see when a baby is growing in a woman's body. However, the mother, during these first three and a half months, may be having morning sickness and feeling different in her body. Likewise, no one sees the changes occurring inside a woman experiencing perimenopause. Hormones are very powerful. They change our bodies through all of these transitions and even at birthing, pushing babies out!

I just hate it when men think PMS is all in our heads. I'd like to see a man have a period and not cry or get angry. Would he be able to carry on life as usual? No! Ladies, perimenopause is real—and it is not your fault! It happens to you because you are a human being who happens to be female. It is also very hard work.

Remember what it was like as a teenager? Were you moody? Did you need more sleep, eat a lot, or feel lazy? Were you unmotivated and cranky? Did you even feel lost at times? Hormonal changes come with symptoms. Unless you know what those symptoms are, you will be in the dark, as I was. Hormones are changing your body to not be fertile anymore and to usher you into the second half of your life. They don't affect you only physically, but also mentally, emotionally, and spiritually. Not an easy task!

Uniqueness

This transition is unique to each woman. Not all women experience the same symptoms and to the same degree. Also, what helps one woman may not help another. Some women have had only one hot flash, and some still have hot flashes into their nineties. I call it a hormonal "grab bag." Every day can be different—and it is different for every woman. I have spoken with lots of women about their experiences, and they are all different. Some breeze right through it and some don't.

One of my favorite books is *Embracing Menopause Naturally* by Gabriele Kushi. She includes stories of women who have gone through the change. It was very helpful and comforting to read about their journeys; my feelings were validated, and I didn't feel so alone. I felt strengthened and empowered from a sense of community with these women. I felt *normal!* This is a normal phase in a woman's life, and whatever I experience is normal for my body. The good news for you is that you are not alone! In this book, I will share many of the symptoms of perimenopause, how to adjust to them, things you can do to ease them, and—for the ones you can't ease—how to make them bearable.

IT CERTAINLY IS A CHANGE!

As a child, you spent most of your time focusing on *yourself.* During adolescence, you changed into a woman. You most likely married, had children, and spent so much time caring for your family, managing a home, and working, that you had little time left for yourself. Not too many years later, you now experience (or will experience) your body going through the momentous change of perimenopause. Then, in your forties and fifties, with the changes in your family and home dynamics, you discover (or will discover) that you have lots of time for *you* again. It definitely is head spinning!

CHAPTER 2

The Symptoms

 c/o

WHEN I WAS YOUNGER, I only knew two things about menopause: some women experienced hot flashes, and eventually, my period would end. I never, in a million years, thought I would have hot flashes. I always thought, "I won't have any of that stuff! That's just for *other* people. It wouldn't happen to me because I always took care of myself, stayed positive, and had faith in God. Was I in for a surprise! "Welcome to the human race, Karen. You are a woman. You have hormones. You will go through the change." I even asked God many times to make it be over—now, please! My prayers went unanswered.

When I started reading books on perimenopause, I really connected with the women who were telling me their symptoms and how they were feeling. I hung onto their words like a lifeline. I knew what I was going through was real, and I wasn't the only one. I discovered it was normal. I didn't like it, but I knew I would make it because these women did, and they told me I would.

Fluctuating hormones impact you emotionally, physically, and psychologically. Estrogen and progesterone have contrasting physiological effects on the body and mind. Since your hormones can fluctuate many times in a day—never mind just in an hour—your symptoms will do the same. Riding the waves of emotions is challenging to say the least. Knowing what is happening is the first key to dealing with it. If you know you may be all over the map, you can recognize it and handle it with some sense of control. You may not have complete control of your hormones, but you can be aware. Knowing what is going on is *everything* to keeping you sane!

The following link shows a chart to the contrasting effects of estrogen and progesterone. It is helpful to know what symptoms will accompany the fluctuating hormones. You will know why you are feeling and acting a certain way. It is also helpful to know which supplements or creams you may need.

http://www.johnleemd.com/physiological-effects-estrogen-progesterone.html

Emotional Symptoms

My emotional symptoms arrived first—at approximately age forty-two. About six years later, I started skipping periods. My periods ended at age fifty and the hot flashes began right after. At least I knew what PMS was and how it affected me; since I didn't know I was in perimenopause, I just thought I was *losing my marbles*.

Feeling out of control

Because of my hormones fluctuating so often, I felt out of control. It seemed that emotions came and went of their own free will, thoughts flew in and out of my mind, and physically I felt like I was falling apart at the seams. "Calgon, take me away!"

Crying

Putting on my coat as I was heading off to work, I'd burst into tears. I had no idea why I was crying. A few times, when I attended my weekly Bible class, I felt very emotional and looked like I was about to cry. My friends asked me how I was doing—I didn't know what was wrong with me or why I was about to fall apart. I just put my head down and tried to be invisible. One lady asked if she could give me a hug; I begged her not to. I knew I would start bawling, and I couldn't explain why. It was so embarrassing.

Self-Doubt

I would be around people at social gatherings and would keep asking my husband, "Am I acting right? Am I saying stupid things?" He reassured me I was acting perfectly fine.

Not Feeling like Myself Anymore

I didn't know who else I was, but I didn't feel like myself! I would walk by the mirror, see myself, and think, "Who is that?"

Feeling Lost, out of Place

I didn't feel like I belonged where I was. I felt like my life was somewhere else, and I had to go find it. It was as if I had amnesia and was searching for my real life.

One thing that gave me comfort was watching the 1970s show *The Waltons*. In one episode, Olivia Walton, who played the mother, was experiencing the upheavals caused by perimenopause. In a letter to John Boy, she wrote, "If I don't find something to hold onto, I feel I'll fly off the world." Watching it, I knew exactly how she felt.

Wanting to Go Home

I just wanted to go home! The only problem was—home wasn't there anymore. I was a grown-up. I wanted to be a little girl again and have someone take care of me. I didn't want to be an adult.

Wanting to Run Away

I kept telling my husband I wanted to run away. I had to go somewhere, but I didn't know where. I just wanted to run!

Depression

I stopped smiling and laughing for such a long time. I was never depressed like this before, so it was an eye opener. Every once in a while, something would make me laugh, and when I did, I realized how long it had been since I had laughed. I didn't want to kill myself; I just didn't want to live anymore! That's how I describe the hard days—I just wanted a long break! I knew exercise helped with depression, but I was not in the mood for seeing people, or jumping around to happy music! All I wanted to do was cry and be left alone until everything was all right again.

Overwhelmed

I felt overwhelmed by everything. I kept saying, "This is too much!" Cooking dinner, doing laundry, and paying bills was all too much. At times, I felt immobilized when I thought of all the things I had to do.

Never having been a messy person, I started leaving my clothes on the floor. I called them my "menapiles." It was too much to put them away. I only did what absolutely needed to be done. I would walk through the house, see the projects I had to do, and just look the other way. The change going on inside me felt so big, I had no mental or physical energy for anything else.

Anger/Rage

I was angry. I didn't like feeling overwhelmed and out of control. I was mad at my husband, just because he was there. I was mad that I couldn't sleep, that I had to get up, and that I was tired. I would holler at people on the phone when I had to call cable or the electric company. Then I would cry and feel like a terrible person. I would scream at my computer, or at people from my past that were long gone. It was exhausting. I lived in my head so much, that it seemed I had no life outside of it.

Making Decisions

Since I didn't know how I would be feeling from minute to minute, making a decision was almost impossible.

Anxiety

I didn't know what anxiety was until perimenopause. It was an awful feeling of fear or a sense of doom in my body, but I didn't know why it was there. I found myself having a drink or two in the middle of the day to take the edge off. I couldn't believe I was drinking! There was no obvious reason for the anxiety, since I was not afraid or nervous about anything. It was just *there*. I called it "body anxiety."

The Past

On Sunday mornings, my husband and I would sit on the porch and watch the birds at the feeder. He would listen to me go on and on with all my stories about when I was a child. I would always end up mad and crying about something or about someone who had hurt me. I decided it was time to face the past and deal with it, so I started going to counseling/therapy, reading books on emotional healing, journaling, and attended Al-Anon. I also had a strong desire to reconnect with people from my past.

Regret/Reflection on My Life

I regretted not doing things I thought I should have done by this time in my life. I regretted the things I did wrong and the mistakes I had made.

Empty Nest

I didn't like that my house had become so quiet—I missed being a mom; I missed the joy of it and the fun I'd had with my son. I wanted it all back.

Grieving

I admit I didn't want to go through this change. Being a mom was wonderful, and I always wanted another baby, so I was sad.

Isolation

I stopped answering the phone and the door. If someone came to the house, I panicked. I didn't want to see or deal with anyone. I would think, "Just go away and leave me alone!" One day, there was a man in a big truck in my driveway, dropping off materials for my husband. I didn't answer the door. He knew I was home, so he called me to convince me he was legitimate—it was quite embarrassing, but he was understanding and said his wife did the same thing.

MENTAL SYMPTOMS

Mentally, I was so overwhelmed that I took a six-year pause in writing this book. I'm back, so there is hope!

Cobwebs

Strange but true, I felt like I had cobwebs in my head. I would feel something in my head and try to shake it out. "Now, I know I am nuts!"

Forgetful

I would be talking and in the middle of the sentence, forget what I was talking about! I had to ask my friend what I was saying to her. While writing an article, the words just fell out of my head; I couldn't remember them for the life of me. (The funny thing was I was going to write about perimenopause!)

I also would have to stop because I couldn't think of simple words. "You know what I'm talking about? The *thing* you put in your mouth to clean your teeth—with the paste on it? It's on the...the white *thing* in the bathroom where water comes out of!" Nowadays, I still talk like this. I have trouble getting words to come out of my mouth. People look at me like I am strange, except other women my age. Then you laugh with me. You should see two perimenopausal women talking to each other. They use the word *thing* a lot.

Tolerating People

I am challenged with dealing with people at this stage of life; for example, when I tell the telephone company my new address for the twenty-fifth time, yet they send my bill to my old address! Really? I am not alone with this one. Many women I talk to say the same thing. Like them, I feel that I *used to* be a nice person.

Controlling Thoughts

My thoughts were all over the place, and it was very challenging to control them. I had some really off-the-wall thoughts pop into my head—I won't even say what they were! That was also a very common symptom among the ladies with whom I spoke. It felt like I was out of control in my head. (Mrs. Walton said the same thing.)

PHYSICAL SYMPTOMS

Loss of Energy

I was always tired and felt heavy. I would wake up exhausted. It seemed like a marathon just to walk downstairs, never mind make breakfast. I would often think, "Ugh! Another day! Can everyone just pretend I'm not here?" I just wanted to walk around in my pajamas, sit in front of the TV, eat, sleep, and talk on the phone with my friends.

Sleep Difficulties/Insomnia/Needing More Sleep

At age forty-nine, I started waking up between 3:00 and 5:00 a.m. and lie there wide awake. It took me hours to fall back asleep, and, of course, I would start to nod off ten minutes before the alarm. Then, I'd have the "sleep coma" when I got up. What a wonderful way to start the day. People say menopausal women are crabby. How crabby would you be if you didn't get a full night's sleep in seven years?

Just as in adolescence, I need more sleep these days. Waking up every night doesn't help! This inside work takes a lot of energy.

Wearing Jewelry

I no longer wanted to wear jewelry. Rings didn't feel comfortable on my fingers anymore and since I was sad, I felt like wearing earrings and necklaces were only for happy times.

Hot Flashes and Night Sweats

They were kind of funny at first. "Oh hon, I'm having a warm flash!" I'd laugh and fan my face proudly while drinking my tea. When the warmth turned to hot flashes, I found myself running outside in the dead of winter and thinking, "Wow, is it *nice* out here," as the wind and snow were pelting my face. I spent a lot of time taking my sweater off and putting it back on.

It is different for every woman, but for me, there was a panicky, anxious feeling when the hot flash first began. I would feel an uncomfortable sense of energy coming out of nowhere, and then a feeling of impending doom, like something bad was about to happen. I instantly craved something sweet; bowls of ice cream passed before my eyes. Right now, a drink would be nice to stop the anxiety. I would get so hot I thought I was going to explode and I wanted to be left alone. I didn't want anyone to talk to me, ask me for anything, or touch me until it was over. It is really easy to fly off the handle during them. My husband knew when one was starting, because my face became red, and afterward, I had a layer of glistening sweat on my face.

Hot flashes are pretty distracting, and it is challenging to get through a situation involving other people, especially if you are trying to look professional. At public speaking events, I would warn people what I was going through beforehand. I didn't want them wondering why I was fanning myself and spritzing my face with water.

Another time, I was in the grocery store when I felt both a hot flash and a sneeze about to erupt. I have learned that if I don't cross my legs when I sneeze, I will surely be changing my pants. I must have been quite a sight—ripping off my coat and sweater and crossing my legs at the same time.

A hot flash is similar to a labor contraction. The contraction begins, reaches its peak, then starts to subside. Both activities require breathing to manage them.

When night sweats would occur, which are just hot flashes in the night, my arms and legs would search for the cold spots on the sheets, and I would flip my pillow over because it's always cooler on the other side. I'd turn the fan on, throw off the covers, and sometimes I'd have to sit up. They usually happened between three and six a.m. When I first started having them, I really soaked the sheets. Then I would have to wake my husband so we could change the bed.

During my first year of having hot flashes, I would think, *"Another* one?" I got so annoyed by them. I had no idea that once they started, they would keep coming! I didn't know how permanent and bothersome they would be. I have since figured out that I have averaged about thirty-five hot flashes a day. Multiply this by 365 days, then by six years, (because I was hot

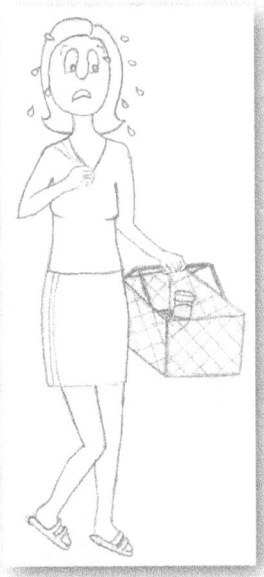

Picture by Abbie Moschell

flash-free for one year), and the grand total of hot flashes I have had is 76,650! I figure I spent about four minutes dealing with each one: I would have to get up, turn on the fan or run outside, take off my sweater, breathe through it all, put my sweater back on, come back in the house or turn the fan off, and resume what I was doing. I figured out that I spent about two hours and twenty minutes a day just dealing with hot flashes. (And I am still having them!)

Speak of the devil, here's one now. Even my glasses are too hot to keep on my face! I am very aware of the knee socks I have on and these hot jeans! Off goes the sweater and I am out the door! Okay, I am freezing now; time to go back in.

Irregular Periods/Heavy, Long Ones

I skipped periods on and off for two years, and then the last one lasted for two months with very heavy bleeding. It left me very anemic. I was munching on ice chips day and night for weeks!

Migraines
Although some women suffer from them, I didn't experience the joy of migraines, thank God!

Digestive Problems
Some women have digestive problems at this time, because as we get older, we have less hydrochloric acid to digest food. Also, the state of our stomachs reflects the state of our hearts and minds. If you are upset or pulled in too many directions, your stomach will not be at ease.

Constipation
I remember I was always constipated for the first few days of my period and pregnancy was no picnic either. It seemed no matter how healthy I ate, I struggled with constipation when perimenopause started. During this time, I ate vegetarian, vegan, raw, meat, drank lots of water, exercised, but nothing seemed to help. I would have to take a natural supplement every few weeks to help depending on the need. (Good news: when the hot flashes reduced, so did the constipation).

Stiffness/Achy Joints
I started feeling like I was all thumbs and my hands didn't work as well. It is also a little harder to get up after sitting in one position for a while.

A Little Extra Weight in the Belly
Again, due to the effect of too much estrogen from lack of progesterone, it is easier to gain weight in your midsection. This is compounded with eating too much when we are emotionally stressed.

Changes in sex drive

What happened to my sex drive? There were times when I was not interested at all and it was just a chore and then times when I thought I was twenty-one again!

Vaginal Dryness

I didn't think this would happen either. Intercourse just got a little tricky.

Heart Palpitations

My heart would start pumping really fast. I noticed it, got a little nervous, and before I knew it, it was over. I thought I had imagined it.

Low Thyroid

Many women have thyroid issues at this time in their lives. (See chapter 4 for a resource to help with this issue.)

Thinning Hair

It is normal to lose about one hundred hairs a day. I remember washing my hair and seeing a little extra in the drain. It wasn't for very long, and then it went back to the normal amount.

Comfort

All I wanted was to be comfortable and have no stress. I wanted to stop the world so I could catch up. I didn't want to do errands or any housework. I didn't want to talk to anyone or answer the phone. I thought "Please just leave me alone."

SPIRITUAL SYMPTOMS

As in adolescence, I began to question my faith. I started doubting my beliefs. It was such a difficult time for me, and I wondered if God was really there. I was mad at Him for creating menopause. I also would call out to Him at night and accuse Him of being asleep—since I wasn't!

THE LADIES SHARE

Laura said, "I don't tolerate people anymore. I see a little inkling of myself sometimes. I don't want to do anything—too much, overwhelmed. I don't want any more responsibility. Simple, simple, simple!"

Pam said, "At times, usually when I am in some type of gathering, it's like having my own personal summer. I can feel the hot flash beginning around my shoulders, moving up my neck, my face, then down my body. I start to sweat everywhere, and then it looks like my head is going to explode as my face and ears become as red as an apple. At this point, I can feel it [the heat] in my hair. I am not sure which is more troublesome, the crankiness, the lack of energy, the hot flashes, the lost feelings, or when I need to go—I need to go now!"

Monica said, "Pretty uneventful, sporadic periods for about six months, sometimes very heavy, then no periods for the past year or so. I had very minimal hot flashes—two to five per day."

Adrian said, "Not really sure I've had symptoms other than a couple of night sweats, but even those weren't like the stories I've heard. They didn't even soak the sheets, just my neck. My periods are irregular, and I can't tell if I'll ever have another."

Terri said, "It has been twelve years since I started perimenopause. Just the normal night sweats, hot flashes, and sleepless nights. I took an herbal combination called Flash Fighters that helped immensely. A couple of nights I would get out of bed, take a cold shower, and sit naked in the office playing *Spider Solitaire* because I couldn't sleep. I would be in the grocery store checkout and would get so hot that I wanted to rip my clothes off right there!"

Kathy said, "Was having hot flashes and night sweats along with digestion problems for a year or more and couldn't get a good night's sleep, which
resulted in a foggy head. I started taking Progest at the recommendation of
my chiropractor. The hot flashes and night sweats disappeared—so did the
fogginess in my head. Found out I have quite a number of food allergies.
Paying attention to what I eat has alleviated digestion problems considerably.
I do still have memory lapses occasionally."

Jean said, "I did not like what you said, Karen, when I told you how I was
feeling lately, and you said it was perimenopause. I did not want to accept it,
but I think that's it."

Holly said, "I get hot flashes during my bubble baths."

Elinor said, "I had one hot flash, and that was it."

Samantha said, "I felt like I had dementia. My last period was at age forty-
six. At age forty-eight, I was looking for some hormones. I couldn't sleep or
think. Give me something! I started taking HRT, and I got me back."

CHAPTER 3

Your Tool Bag

༄

Breathe. You're going to be okay. Breathe and remember that
you've been in this place before. You've been this uncomfortable
and anxious and scared, and you've survived. Breathe and
know that you can survive this too. These feelings can't break
you. They're painful and debilitating, but you can sit with
them and eventually, they will pass. Maybe not immediately,
but sometime soon, they are going to fade and when they do,
you'll look back at this moment and laugh for having doubted
your resilience. I know it feels unbearable right now, but keep
breathing, again and again. This will pass. I promise it will pass.

—Daniell Koepke

Read and Learn

Learning about perimenopause is at the top of the list! It will arm you with knowledge that will calm your fears by letting you know what is happening in your mind and body. Don't try to live your life as though you are in your thirties. Life is different now, and things are changing—whether you like it or not. Adjust the best you can. Here are some books that helped me immensely:

The Wisdom of Menopause, by Christiane Northrup, MD
Embracing Menopause Naturally, by Gabriele Kushi
The Silent Passage by Gail Sheehy

Now, here comes some honesty: I know that every woman has a different experience with perimenopause. Some women breeze right through it, and others have a harder time. I know I was pretty darn challenged. Where my experience lies on the charts, I am not sure. I can only go by how I felt on whether it was a little difficult or a lot. *It was a lot difficult.*

As I mentioned, I was in pretty good physical shape, ate organic, whole foods, didn't smoke, and was a positive-thinking, spiritual person. I took the suggestions I read about for symptoms of perimenopause, but I learned that not every herb or supplement will work the same for every woman. I tried many natural treatments and most just worked a little or temporarily. In the case of the hot flashes, with all the treatments I tried, I still have them, but they are milder and less often. I am not sure if that is the supplement or my hormones just leveling out with time. I am telling you this so you don't become frustrated if something doesn't work for you. The label on the bottles will say they make hot flashes go away but that is not always the case. You can have your hormone levels tested to see, more accurately, what you may need to reduce symptoms. I did once, but didn't keep up with the testing because I was too overwhelmed.

When I was pregnant, I wanted to have a natural birth; I did not want drugs. Then the labor started. I did not realize how challenging it was going to be, so I ended up taking something to take the edge off the pain. The same goes with the symptoms of perimenopause. You can go through them without any hormones, supplements, or help of any kind. Many women do. It all depends on how many symptoms you have and their severity. When my hot flashes came, they were so uncomfortable and were such an interruption in my life, I knew I had to get something to help. The emotional turmoil became too much, so I went to therapy. When the anxiety became too much, I took supplements for it. When I started walking around like a zombie from insomnia, I took something natural to help me sleep. I still needed to function in my life.

Every day is different, and I must deal with whatever I am handed. We can do things to ease the symptoms, but can we really erase them? If I am in labor, I can take something to ease the labor pains, but can I stop them? If I am depressed, I can take an antidepressant but will that make all the challenges in my life go away? I am aging. I may do things to make myself look younger or be healthier, but I am still aging!

When I have hot flashes, I must breathe through them until they pass. I must accept the fact that they are there until they leave and no one can tell me when they will end. I can only educate myself, get support, and adjust my lifestyle during this time. I can only try to be as blessed as I can through it all. I can trust God to hold my hand through this transition. I have a wooden sign in my kitchen that says:

> *God doesn't give us what we can handle; God helps us handle what we've been given.*

Sometimes life can be rough, and we wonder why—since we have faith in God. I was under the impression that faith in God meant things would always be great. Well, yes, they can be great, but there is another side to the coin. My Bible-scholar friend wrote an article called "Suffering Well." Here is a paragraph from the article and the link to the full article, if you would like to read the rest of it. It is not about hormones but rather how to deal with the difficulties of life that we all experience:

> Often Christians have an expectation that because God loves them, or because they have faith, their life will be easy, or at least easier than other people's lives. Many Christians expect a "blessed" life, but what they usually mean by that is a "problem-free life," something that the Bible never promises. Actually, it is just the opposite. God promises us there will be problems in this life, and not to be surprised by that. "Beloved, do not be surprised at the fiery trial when it comes upon you to test you, as though something strange were happening to you. (1 Pet. 4:12 ESV)

The link is http://www.truthortradition.com/articles/suffering-well.

GET SUPPORT

Caution—do not go down this road alone!

We were not designed to handle life all by ourselves. If you are having a hard time with the change, do not do it by yourself! On a regular basis, talk to someone you can trust and who is not judgmental about how you feel. Don't let things build up till you are ready to commit yourself to a mental institution. It is good to have someone to share with, what you are experiencing.

Be around people. Don't isolate for too long. If you are a stay-at-home mom, plan a play date for yourself. Connecting with people early in the day is helpful. Make it a practice to call a friend in the morning if you can. Find a balance between time alone with self-care and socializing with others and service.

Plan to go shopping with a friend—that way you don't sit home dreading the trip.

Get a walking partner. Go outside and walk down the road for seven minutes. You have to walk back, so you will have walked about a mile.

A FEW WORDS ABOUT A WOMAN'S LIFE

Multitasking is common for women. We care for our homes and our families; we have jobs, aging parents, and so forth. *The typical woman—servant to all!* I had to cope with a variety of settings because of my diverse work background. I am mostly self-employed, so I work from my home and also take jobs outside of my home. I can appreciate the stress for both realms. In addition, I took care of my aging mom and father-in-law. I also have a granddaughter, so I spend lots of time with her. My husband has his own business, so I help out with that. I have a massage therapy and health-coaching business. We take individuals into our home at times. I had a job outside of the home with the elderly, and I volunteer. The struggle for women is to keep going during perimenopause while living life, working a job, and serving others. Something's got to give!

At times, I backed off from working, because it all became too much for me. I was able to work less, but staying home had its own challenges. Although I liked being in my comfort zone, it was easier to give in to my feelings, because I was alone. I didn't have face-to-face contact with many people. I felt myself becoming a "homebody." I didn't want to go places, because I was too comfortable right where I was. I became lonely and was in my head too much.

When I started working again, I had to prepare myself mentally because of being overwhelmed. Although, once I got out the door, I felt energized by moving and being with people. The human interactions were the best! I would look back and think "Oh Karen, you have to have a job and not stay home." It was much easier when I was out with others.

Working and trying to be professional during perimenopause was a challenge. I would have clients in front of me, and while listening to them, I'd be sweating and fanning myself. It was quite embarrassing. They told me not to worry about it, but I didn't like it.

I worked at an assisted living home and realized that there were many women co-workers who were having hot flashes, so I fit right in. There were fans there, so I was all set—except for in the tub room. I was assisting the elderly with their baths; they had a Jacuzzi tub so when they turned on the bubbles, I melted. I would sit on the tile floor where it was cooler. I felt like a dog!

The activity room was always seventy-two degrees and very sunny. During activities, I always had a fan blowing on me. The residents would laugh and ask, "Are you still having those hot flashes?"

Twice a year I travel to a resort where I massage ladies for three days straight. Once I was so tired from not sleeping at night that I cried silently while giving a massage. You know, when you get to that point of exhaustion, all that you can do is laugh or cry. I got through it, but it was rough.

When I worked from home, there were times that I had so much anxiety that I drank a few glasses of wine around lunch time. One day I remembered I had a massage to give later that afternoon. The stress of the pressure to get myself together and do my job was overwhelming. I pulled it together, though, and got it done. Yes, it was rough.

My husband and I would play guitars and sing for the elderly and at church events. I would get a hot flash while singing; they were so distracting, and I felt like everyone could tell. Oh, my! Could I just be a man for a while?

Learn to ask for help at home and at work. Other people can't read your mind, so ask specifically for what you need. Tell your boss you are going through the change. Since they hire humans to work for them, they will most likely understand. Take a crying break in the bathroom if you need it. When you get home, take some time alone for a few minutes if you can. Explain the change to your teenagers. They will understand because it is a lot like what they are going through. It can be a great bonding time with them.

Share with your spouse or partner what you are learning about perimenopause. This will help your beloved to be more informed and compassionate. Mine was (although I did drive him a little crazy).

A FEW WORDS FOR SPOUSES/PARTNERS

Depending on the severity of symptoms, the "other half" can get pummeled during this time. Partners, you are going through the change too. It does put stress on the relationship. Women, like men, seek understanding. Read and learn about what your partner is experiencing. It isn't all in her head; it is real and challenging for her. The change is very hard inside work. Even though you can't see it, it is monumental, like a pregnancy. Try to remember your adolescence. You didn't want to be grouchy to those around you, but you were, at times. You felt lost, while your body was doing its own thing. Compassion will go a long way to help her deal with her symptoms. Talking with her regularly will help her release some of the buildup of emotional steam. You don't have to say much, just listen.

Go see *Menopause the Musical* with her. Watch the movie *Fried Green Tomatoes*, and read the books I recommended at the beginning of this chapter.

Find common ground to stay together during this time. Lots of couples divorce, because it can be so challenging. My husband and I have our faith and granddaughter. We both survived it. The change won't last forever, so work hard to stay together.

Living with a woman going through the change will teach you how to love bigger. She will be very grateful for this. Women would like you to read their minds and know what they need. We know this is not possible. Sometimes it is hard for a woman to ask for help because of the emotions she is dealing with. It would be a great help to her if you asked her what she needs. I think God has special rewards for you partners, as you love her through this. Be survivors together. It gets better.

Emotional Help

Try not to focus on your feelings too much. I know it is challenging, and I didn't always do this very well. What is "doing well"? I guess I felt that if I allowed myself to get depressed, it was bad. Was it? Maybe I could stop judging things. Maybe I could cut myself a break and just do the best I could. Looking back, I would say, "Love yourself, and try to keep as happy as you can." I am so glad perimenopause is over, and my hormones are much more stable. I never did like the rollercoaster!

Don't try to be perfect. Sometimes just do "good enough." Some days, you will get nothing done that you had planned. It's okay. If you were sick, you would take days off. Perimenopause is not an illness, but with hormones racing up and down, you may feel out of control emotionally. Until your hormones become more stable, you need to cut yourself some slack. You may still have to go to your job, do the dishes, and make supper, but have compassion for yourself.

It just felt so strange to me how I compared this to being sick. It felt ridiculous that going through perimenopause took so much of my energy. It set me back with my everyday work and goals. Friends would ask me to help them with something, and I had to decline because all I wanted to do was stay home where I was comfortable and safe. It was too much. I was asked to join a business with two licensed counselors, but I just couldn't get myself together. One of the counselors (a man) said to me, "You can do it if you think you can." I knew that, but I really didn't think I could. I didn't know what would be in the hormonal grab bag every morning. If it were anxiety, it would not be a good day. I decided I didn't want the pressure to try to move past it. It was challenging enough to make supper, never mind to speak in front of clients.

Don't ask your emotions if they want to do something. Leave them out of it. If you need to go to the grocery store, just go.

There are two people you may want to eliminate from your life. Their names are Mr. & Mrs. Should. Do things because you *want to* not because you *should*. Their voices will cause pressure and guilt. Try rewording your chores such as "I want to clean my kitchen," instead of, "I should clean my kitchen." Saying "I want to go for a walk," makes it fun instead of the guilt ridden statement, "I should go for a walk."

Make a plan for tomorrow so you can be productive, but don't plan too much because you may become overwhelmed. Space out your chores and errands, so you get a break.

Remember perimenopause is temporary. Keep telling yourself this. Write it on paper and tape it on your kitchen cabinets.

Stay grateful. Focus on what you have. Look at all your blessings; this really helps.

Your own words are stronger and have more influence on yourself than anyone else's. Do you know that this is true? Try coaching yourself through a situation, and see how powerful your words are. "Okay, Karen, you can do this. You will be okay; just breathe. It feels very difficult right now, but you will make it through this moment. It won't last forever." This way, you can have your best friend with you all the time. Get good at validating your feelings and reaffirming yourself. Write in a journal things that you can say to yourself. Write them on your hand if you need to. You will heed your own words.

Help someone who is in need. The recipient of your kindness will be most grateful, and you will feel wonderful. Also, your kindness distracts you from the emotional roller coaster that you are riding, which is a double blessing for you!

Crying/Feelings

If you feel like crying, just let it out! When I would become emotional, I held it in. I was afraid that if I started crying, I wouldn't stop. Going to Al-Anon gave me a new perspective on that. When it was my turn to speak at a meeting, no one said anything. I was allowed to express my feelings with no comments or judgements. No one told me I shouldn't feel the way I did. I started allowing myself to feel whatever I was feeling and let the tears roll. I would say to myself, "it is okay to be you, Karen. Your feelings are important, and you have a reason to cry, so go ahead." It was very liberating to let myself feel and I discovered I didn't cry forever. Do you remember being told as kids that we had nothing to cry about? Well, we really did and holding it in didn't make it go away.

Remember that your feelings are *your* feelings. If someone physically hurts or insults you, you know how you feel. When someone tells you that you shouldn't feel the way you feel, think about how silly that is. How can anyone tell you how to feel? If I am sad or happy, I know it. If I am miserable, I take a minute and figure out what I need. Denying how you feel is not mentally healthy. Also, know that not everything you feel is actually the truth. For example, if I run into people I know at the grocery store, on a very emotional day, will it really be "the worst"? I also may feel I am losing my mind at times, but is that the truth? Remember that feelings are not final and they change frequently. Sit with them for a few minutes, acknowledge them, and let them drift away.

PHYSICAL TIPS

Hot Flash Help

Dress in layers, so you can adjust yourself according to how hot you become. That way you aren't tempted to rip all your clothes off in public!

If you have a hot flash at the market, rush to the frozen section quickly. Open the door and pretend you are looking over the frozen foods.

Once, while grocery shopping, I commented to the checkout girl that I always have a hot flash when it comes time to pay for my food. She told me that it is always warmer up front at the registers. Now I think ahead and remove my jacket before I arrive there. As a result, I am not in a panic to escape!

Do not suffer. The heat from hot flashes can be overwhelming. Moving air made me able to get through them. Bring a fan with you wherever you go, and put one in every room of your house. I have a small fan in my kitchen, one at my desk (with special rocks to hold down my papers), one in the living room right near where I sit on the couch, and one on a small table near my bed, so I can reach it easily. Wherever I go, I sit near an outlet to plug in my fan.

When I visit at a friend's house, I choose the chair near a window or the door in case I need to run outside to the cool air quickly. At large meetings, I sit at the end of the row of chairs. This helps, because sometimes I feel claustrophobic when I am sitting in a crowd, and that triggers hot flashes.

Put a few drops of peppermint oil in a spray bottle with water to mist your skin—peppermint is very cooling. Then, fan yourself with a cardboard paint chart from the paint store. It fits nicely in your purse.

To cool off during a hot flash, let cold water run over your wrists at the sink. (I did that when I was pregnant.) While driving, I stick one arm out of the window. The cold air on my skin distracts me from feeling the heat. When my husband drives, I stick my head out.

Putting a bath towel on the bed sheet before you go to sleep is a good idea. If you have a night sweat, you can just remove the towel and lay back down on a dry sheet. The only problem will be the top sheet. I usually just deal with it being a little moist. (I haven't figured that part out yet.)

Breathe through hot flashes. Try the 4-7-8 breathing exercise. This is very helpful for anxiety: close your eyes, inhale for four seconds through your nose. Hold it for seven seconds. Blow out your breath for eight seconds. You cannot be anxious while you are breathing deeply. This was very helpful for me.

Keep your house cool. I would rather wear a sweater than have a hot flash triggered by too much warmth.

Find out what triggers your hot flashes; they are different for everyone. Mine are the first sip of a cup of hot tea, a glass of wine, eating foods with too much sugar, being too warm, feeling claustrophobic, getting upset over something, sleeping, and breathing! Sometimes they make sense, and sometimes they don't. Hot flashes are nice when I go to the ocean. Since

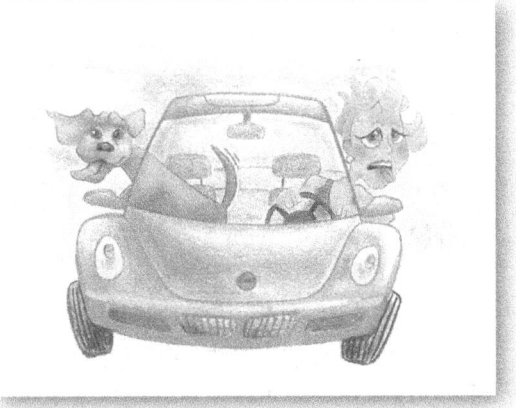

Picture by Becky Staneruck

the water is usually cold, I wait for a hot flash, and then I run in. All I feel is total refreshment. Two minutes later, I am bolting out!

Get more sleep. Take naps. Close your eyes for five minutes after lunch.

For vaginal dryness during intimacy, use coconut oil for lubrication and proceed slowly.

Try going outside every day. Get fresh air and sit in the sunshine. Let the sun produce some nice vitamin D on your skin. In addition, you will be making serotonin, which will help you feel emotionally better, and melatonin, which will help you sleep. Take off your shoes and walk around on the grass barefoot.

Exercise like a child—do fun things!

Kids don't exercise; they just keep moving, and they only do what's fun. You may not feel like exercising, so don't! I put on some 70s music, and I dance around my kitchen. While talking on the phone, I walk around my driveway and yard. I keep a five-pound weight on my desk and work my biceps a few times a day. While waiting for food to cook, I bend over and stretch my spine, and that leads me to do other stretches; then I may do three squats. While watching TV, I stretch my calves. If thinking you have to have a thirty-minute exercise routine every day, think again.

Put a rebounder in your living room, and jump ten times when you walk past it. While dancing, throw in a few jumping jacks. Get a book about stretching, and put it on your coffee table. When you are watching a movie, get on the floor, and do a few stretches. When you add all of this up, you will have done quite a bit. You need to move, but you don't have to be in shape to run a marathon. You just need to be in shape to live your own life. Remember not to say "I should exercise." Instead say, "I think I will do five jumping jacks and rock out to my favorite music!"

Nourishing activities

Keep in mind that there other things to help you to feel better than just eating carbs.

Find activities that nourish your heart and soul and do those. Here are some suggestions. Make up your own list.

Call a friend and gab for an hour.

Volunteer at a nursing home or assisted living. Offer your time to just listen to them. They have great life stories to tell and they will appreciate your time more than you know.

Get a hug/give a hug.

Read a good book.

Start laughing for no reason at all. Do it around your kids and see how contagious it is!

Watch a girly movie.

Play your favorite music and dance your heart out.

Go for a nature walk.

Sit by the lake or ocean.

Listen to a bible teaching.

Get a massage or give one.

Do things that make you smile and laugh.

Herbs and Supplements to Balance Hormones

There are many herbs and natural supplements that can help to balance hormones and relieve some symptoms. Go to your local health food store and ask for suggestions. They are very helpful and know what is popular with the women. I took a plant supplement called Phyto B by Bezwecken that took my hot flashes away for a year. It was heavenly until my body changed, and my hot flashes came back. Hormones are always changing, so you may need to try different products to address the need of the day.

Magdalena Wszelaki, a certified holistic health coach, is an expert at teaching you to rebalance your hormones with food. She has a hormone quiz you can take to see where your hormones are at.

https://www.hormonesbalance.com/quiz/

Dr. Christiane Northrup offers lots of suggestions on herbs and supplements to help with hot flashes, insomnia, and so forth in her book, *The Wisdom of Menopause.*

Thyroid Issues

If you think you are having thyroid issues, you can check out Andrea Beaman. She is a certified health coach, author of four books, and an expert on the thyroid. Her website is www.AndreaBeaman.com. Type "thyroid health" in the search bar.

A Word about Neurotransmitters

If your neurotransmitters (brain chemicals) are imbalanced, they can lead to or exacerbate hormone imbalances. Some of your brain chemicals are serotonin, GABA, dopamine, epinephrine, and so on. You could have symptoms such as sleeplessness, anxiety, tiredness, lack of energy, cravings, and hot flashes due to amino acid deficiencies. Being low in serotonin can trigger hot flashes. Getting your neurotransmitter levels tested and obtaining products to balance them can help with hormonal symptoms. A naturopathic doctor can order a test for you. If your doctor is educated in this area, he/she may be able to order a test also. I recommend the company NeuroScience. You can check on their website for doctors who offer this service. Their website is https://www.neuroscienceinc.com. Two great resources to help with neurotransmitters are: the book *Female Brain Gone Insane: An Emergency Guide for Women Who Feel like They Are Falling Apart* by Mia Lundin, RNC, NP and two books by Julia Ross, MA; *The Diet Cure* and *The Mood Cure*.

AND FINALLY, THE GOOD THINGS!

The change seemed to bring things up from my past. I had many issues that I didn't know I had. I decided to revisit these issues from my childhood and early adulthood. From the counseling I had received, I learned that our past does affect how we think, feel, and act as adults. I learned to be aware of my feelings and "sit" with them. Many times I would have moments of flashbacks. They would come unexpectedly, triggered by something that had just occurred. Once I got angry at my husband for cooking food on the grill. There was no reason for being mad at him, but I was. I asked God to show me why I was angry. I stayed with the feelings, and soon I connected them with an event that had happened in the past that was similar to the current situation. I was able to work through the moment by discovering where the thinking pattern originated.

Feelings come from thoughts. When we think the same thoughts long enough, they become automatic feelings. You can figure out the thoughts behind the feelings by investigating where they may have first developed. Once I became aware of what I was feeling, I mulled it over until I traced it back to the situation where the thoughts first began. Now, I think about whether those thoughts are right or wrong according to what I believe about myself and change them. I am not a slave to my feelings anymore.

Being a Christian, I was always encouraged to just say that I was fine, no matter if I was or not. There is a balance to speaking positive but it is not healthy to deny everything. It is human to have feelings and it is okay to admit them—this is how you deal with them. Jesus had emotions and he didn't deny them. He wept, got angry, and was exceeding sorrowful before his time of suffering. I am sure he spent much time laughing and being happy too! The change was like an emotional earthquake to me; however, as a result of this experience, I became a healthier person.

In some cultures, women look forward to this time of life because they are revered as being very wise and as a result, have a higher status in their community.

I have gained a greater sense of awareness and have gone through a lot of healing. I have learned that I am as important as anyone else, and that my opinion matters. I stopped thinking that everyone else is smarter than me. I started having more confidence in my ability to make intelligent decisions. If I make a mistake, I remember it isn't the end of the world. I thank the change for all of this. I know that during the times of my greatest struggles, I have grown the most. I am looking forward to the next phase of my life.

It is possible to eventually embrace this experience and treasure it, once you become accustomed to the ride. Unfortunately, this may be almost at its completion. Whatever the case, at the end of your journey, you will have learned much about yourself and discovered a wiser, amazing, beautiful, and revitalized woman!

CHAPTER 4

Eating "Better Than"

ꝏ

YOUR BODY IS VERY SMART. It knows how to heal itself and bring you into a state of balance, given the right ingredients and lifestyle habits. You can ease your symptoms by making simple changes in what you eat. The right foods will help to balance your hormones. Any changes you make toward the better will help. I know this can be challenging to do if you are already overwhelmed. I am a holistic health coach, and it was hard for me too. I did succumb to eating things that made me feel happy at the moment but not in the long run.

Eating *real* foods that have lots of nutrients in them is the key. This does not have to be difficult. Just think of what your grandma would have served you. I know Americans have gotten away from real foods for convenient, boxed and canned foods that can be heated in a microwave. Quick is nice but not always your friend! Foods, slowly prepared with love, are!

As I said, your body is smart. It knows if it needs some protein, some carbs, or some fat. It knows if it wants some fresh fruit or a big salad. When you are hungry, let your body choose, not your eyes. Listen to your body, and ask it what it needs. Just don't go to the fridge and eat whatever is there. Most of my adult life I was either vegetarian or vegan. When I was in perimenopause, my body wanted meat! I was shocked. My husband was sitting there eating a hamburger. I was looking at it and asked, "Can I have a bite?" My body wanted meat protein, so that is what I gave it.

Everyone is the same yet a little different. You may eat foods that I cannot and vice versa. I am sensitive to certain foods, and you may not be. I know what my body likes and what it doesn't. I know if I feel good or not so good after every meal. If I eat a meal and don't feel well afterward, I just say, "Well, I guess I won't eat that again." I can get away with eating some dairy but not too much. Also, the size of my meal is very important to my digestive health. I love food, but I need to be careful not to eat until I am full. I simply eat a little less and I feel so much better. A great book to read is *The Slow Down Diet* by Marc David. Of all the "diet" books I have read, this is at the top of my list. It is about eating for pleasure, energy, and weight loss. It is not your typical diet book. I don't like diet books, as there are too many things I have to change according to "their" rules and I know I won't do it. I would rather listen to my body and do what it says.

Better Than

My motto is "better than." What I mean is, I may not be eating the absolute best thing in the world right now, but it is better than what I could have eaten! Do better than before. Change is not always easy, and you can take baby steps. As long as it is not a life and death decision, you can make a few changes at a time. Habits take time to break, and if you are emotionally overwhelmed, it won't happen. If you keep doing better than, you will eventually be eating great. If you eat two pieces of toast with jelly for breakfast today (lots of sugar), then tomorrow eat one with some almond butter and an egg. If you are drinking two cups of coffee today, then make one of them decaf tomorrow. When I first met my husband, he was putting three teaspoons of white sugar in his coffee! So I would bump his arm and a few grains would fall off the spoon; I told him he would never notice the difference. Now, he has one teaspoon of real maple syrup in his two-thirds decaf organic coffee with organic half and half. He said it was a painless change. Don't overwhelm yourself with changing your menu for the whole week. Just take one meal at a time.

Good Enough

The other motto I love is "good enough." The pressure to be perfect is not healthy! Do not make being perfect your goal. It is exhausting, and you will never attain it anyway.

Keep it simple! You don't have to cook gourmet meals. I don't. If making salad is overwhelming, just serve the vegetables on a plate. Sometimes eating a handful of cashews and some cucumber slices is good enough! And surprisingly, good enough can actually be the best!

I don't keep junk foods in the house, so when I am craving something sweet, I have to be inventive. Sometimes I grab the peanut butter jar and a handful of dates. Or, better yet, I make ice cream in my VitaMix using yogurt, frozen strawberries, and a dab of real maple syrup. Then, I add the homemade chocolate syrup. This takes me literally two minutes to make. Yum! Sometimes I eat popcorn with butter and grated cheese and make myself some homemade "ginger ale." It is tasty enough for me and still better than a bag of candy, and the foods have nutrition in them. Let's face it—I am human. If I am craving to feel better, then sometimes I go to food. It's not like I do it every meal and every day; I try to keep it as healthy as I can.

Starting off the day with a breakfast loaded with sugar will only make your symptoms worse. Remember, refined sugars or foods that turn to sugar, are not your friend! I have more hot flashes the more sugar/carbs I eat. Protein foods with fat like nuts, eggs, and sausage are a good way to start the day. I love a handful of cashews with my green tea or organic coffee. Then I may have an apple and some eggs a little later with one piece of gluten-free toast with butter and almond butter on top. You could also have leftovers from supper.

EAT REAL FOOD

Buy real food and cook it in a pan on the stove—old-fashioned, real food. Your body will choose what it needs from this real food to function correctly.

What is real food? Go to a local farm and see what they are selling that they just pulled out of the ground. Put lots of grass-fed butter on your veggies, and eat locally raised meat. Oh, and after you bake your chicken, eat the skin. Fat is good for you.

Nutrient-dense foods are protein, vegetables, beans, whole grains, fruits, nuts, seeds, and fats. Healthy fats are your friend. They help balance your hormones and keep you satisfied when eating; therefore, you won't overeat. Nuts, nut butters, seeds, grass-fed butter, coconut, and avocados—I eat them often.

DON'T EAT FAKE FOOD

Avoid foods that are low fat, lite, or sugar-free. These foods have fake sugars in them. Sugar-free cookies are made with sugar alcohols. That is not on the healthy list. Make your own cookies from scratch. It's okay to have desserts, but make them yourself and not from a box mix. Use flour, real butter, eggs, and vanilla! They always taste better and are much healthier for you. Since you have to make them and wash the bowls and pans, you won't do it too often.

Tips

Next time you shop, buy two new foods that you will add to your menu.

Whenever you cook, cook extra and save it in the fridge for another meal. Also, freeze some meals so you can have a "cook-free" night!

Most importantly, whatever you eat, enjoy it. Eating food is supposed to be enjoyable! Also, your digestion will be much improved when you have happy emotions while eating.

Again, when you give your body the nutrients and physical movement it needs, it will always try to come into balance and heal itself.

CHAPTER 5

Spiritual Encouragement

❃

GOD LOVES US SO MUCH that He designed our bodies so we wouldn't have babies when we are old. I don't believe God intended for us to suffer during the change. I'm sure Adam and Eve had something to do with it! Trying to handle the difficulties of the change on our own is just too difficult. We can seek His help and confidently rely on Him. He wants to help us through this time. We need to take care of ourselves while being careful not to focus only on our suffering. Turn your thoughts to Him and outward to others. God is wise and kind and He will never leave us alone. He didn't leave Jesus alone and He strengthened him during his suffering.

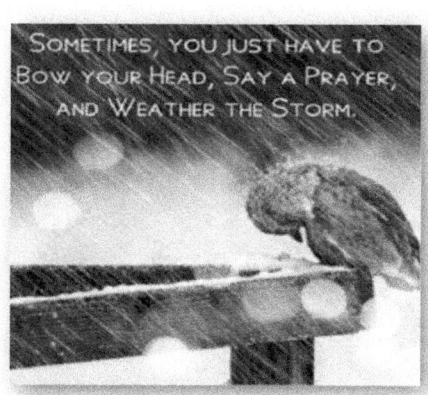

A wonderful quote by LadyCopperRose

Jesus's body was broken, and we can live broken too. I'm sure he was not in the mood to reach out to the man next to him while he was dying. We may not feel good today, but we can still serve others. I don't have to have everything together in my life to bless someone else. Like I said before, don't consult your emotions if you want to do something. Serving is critical to self-care and takes my mind off my pain. Serving helps me! After I quit my job, I began volunteering. I dreaded going, but when I got there, I was able to bless the elderly people. I felt amazing afterward and wondered how I did it. This happened every time; I know God strengthened me in the giving.

God also designed us to be able to focus our minds to be grateful and "suffer well." We all have bodies that don't behave the way we want them to at times. To stay blessed, we can control our thoughts and focus on the right things to get us through each challenge. Jesus had the ability to do it through his ordeal, and so can we. Sometimes I believe I am thinking correctly, but if I am miserable then that is showing me that I am not really in the place in my mind where I could be. Yes, life can and does get really uncomfortable at times, but I can change my thoughts and words to bring me to a thankful and joyful place. If we really, truly, believe what God says in the scriptures, we will be like Jesus was on this earth. We can suffer well and be full of peace and joy. We can live on this earth and be blessed no matter what is going on. It sounds crazy and almost impossible, but "With God all things are possible" (Matt.19:26). He never asks us to do something that we can't do.

We won't be perfect every day or every minute. Nobody can be! Write down on paper, and hang it up, that you are getting off the "perfect" track. I love the quote by Judy Hopps. She said, "Real life is messy." Set your sails toward your destination/goals. The winds and storms will blow you off course. This is a definite guarantee. When you find yourself going off in the wrong direction, reset your sails, and carry on. No guilt, no beating yourself up. This transition may seem like a marathon, and it is a lot of work. Remember to have compassion on yourself. Jesus does.

I know I am so much happier when I am speaking God's words and praising Him. Here is a link to an article about the benefits of praising God:

http://www.chrisheinz.com/read/post/7_benefits_of_praising_god

Watch out for the Quicksand!
There are certain emotions, that when I allow them to stay for too long, I feel myself heading toward a bad place. I can feel myself going downhill and I know I must pull myself out quickly. I know if I allow myself to "go there",

it will be H-E-double hockey sticks! I pray and speak God's Word and there is always a major turnaround.

It is very challenging when my body is in a state of hormonal upheaval. If I keep focusing on my challenges, and whine and complain about them, I am walking right toward the quicksand! My own words and thoughts are dragging me right toward it. Once my feet go into the quicksand, everything escalates. Now, I need the help of someone or something to get me out. I am allowing my emotional thoughts to take over. When I let this happen, I feel desperate and will need to depend on others. People will not always be there for me; they have their own lives and personal challenges to deal with. I must depend on God for help. Fortunately, I can turn to Him and think rightly. Praising God makes it a whole lot easier to stay thankful.

Ladies, we will go through the change either way. God will guide our path when we look to Him. As I said before, I didn't know what was coming, and I was miserable and depressed for a few years until I learned how to handle it. That's why I wrote this book—to help women who are going through the change to have a better experience than I did. Learn from me and other women around you. You can't pray your period or menopause away—I tried that. Educate yourself, learn how to handle the symptoms, get support, stay grateful for what you have, and focus on the promises of God. This will enable you to be more blessed and full of joy, no matter what your body is doing. Remember, this too shall pass.

Hard times, bad times, or tough times, I still have faith in God.

—Andrew Guzaldo

CHAPTER 6

Scriptures to Meditate On

❧

MEDITATING ON SCRIPTURE IS A very powerful healing tool. You can write out verses that are meaningful to you, and put a copy in your purse. No matter where you are, you will always have access to the comforting words from the scriptures.

Proverbs 4:20–23   "My son [daughter], attend to my words; incline thine ear unto my sayings. Let them not depart from thine eyes; keep them in the midst of thine heart. For they are life unto those that find them, and health to all their flesh. Keep thy heart with all diligence; for out of it are the issues of life."
God's words are health to our flesh!

The word *keep* means to guard. Guard your heart with *His* words, and then you won't be blown off course and end up in the quicksand.

Proverbs 17:22   "A merry heart does good like a medicine but a broken spirit dries the bones."

Proverbs 3:5–6   "Trust in the Lord with all your heart and lean not on your own understanding. In all your ways acknowledge Him, and He shall direct your paths."

Titus 2:3–4   "The aged women likewise…that they may teach the young women."

Psalms 18:1–2, 6   "I will love thee, O Lord, my strength. The Lord is my rock, and my fortress, and deliverer; my god, my strength, in whom I will trust; my buckler [a large portable shield that surrounds you on all sides], and the horn of my salvation, and my high tower. In my distress I called upon the Lord and cried unto my God: he heard my voice out of his temple, and my cry came before him, even into his ears."

Psalms 77 is a great book to read in the Bible. At this point, Saul was pursuing David to kill him. David became depressed and overwhelmed. (Who wouldn't?) He was so troubled, that he couldn't even speak. He was thinking that God had abandoned him and the children of Israel. Then David decided to stop focusing on the pain in his soul and reminded himself of all God's wonderful works. He "coached" himself and came back to his right way of thinking—the one of knowing God is there for him and will take care of him. Reading David's words acknowledges my feelings and gives me hope and encouragement.

Psalm 28:4–14   "The Lord is my strength and my shield; my heart trusts
Verse 7   in Him, and I am helped: therefore my heart greatly rejoices; and with my song will I praise Him."
Psalm 27:13–14   Find a Bible and read these verses.
Psalm 35:9   "And my soul shall be joyful in the Lord."
Psalm 42   Please read these eleven verses. The passage ends: "Why art thou cast down, O my soul? And why art thou disquieted within me? Hope thou in God: for I shall yet praise him, who is the health of my countenance, and my God."
Romans 8:18,   I am not alone in suffering and I know God is on my
22–23   side and I am encouraged by His love.

The book of Ephesians simply spells out what God has already done for us. He loves us (2:4) and has quickened (made alive) our mortal bodies (2:1, 5).

He gives us grace to handle what we need to handle (2:5, 8). He strengthens us through the inner man (3:16). He is able to do above and beyond all we can ask or think according to the power that works in us (3:20). What a God we have!

Hebrew 4:15–16	The Lord understands and will give us grace to endure this time.
2 Corinthians 12:8–10	I can rejoice because when I am weak, then am I strong.
Hebrews 13:5	Be content, and know He will never leave you.
1 Peter 5:7	Go fishing! Cast your care on Him.
Philippians 4:6–8	We don't need to be anxious, and we have instructions on what *to* think.
	In light of this verse, "The 4:8 Principle" by Tommy Newberry, is a great book to read.

CHAPTER 7

Journaling
Another Tool for You

THE PURPOSE OF JOURNALING IS self-examination and reflection to reshape/redirect your life.

As a result of journaling, I can see on print, what I am thinking. After I write my thoughts down, I go over them to see what a lie is and what the truth is. Am I telling myself that I am no good or am I reminding myself that I am doing the best I can? Do I speak God's truth to my heart or do I tear myself down?

Here are two links to websites on the benefits of journaling:

https://www.cru.org/train-and-grow/spiritual-growth/devotionals/why-every-christian-should-keep-a-journal.html

http://psychcentral.com/lib/the-health-benefits-of-journaling/

What am I grateful for today?

_____

_____

_____

_____

How am I feeling right now?

_____

_____

_____

What physical symptoms did I have today?

_____

_____

_____

What can I do to help myself feel better physically?

_____

_____

_____

Scriptures I can meditate on today...

_____

_____

_____

Things I did to rest today...

_____

_____

_____

Ways I asked for help today...

_____

_____

_____

What fun exercise did I do today?

_____

_____

_____

What I heard today from the holy spirit?

_____

_____

_____

What are three things that I love about myself?

_____

_____

_____

How did I love today in spite of my feelings?

_____

_____

_____

CHAPTER 8

Words to Myself

❦

I will say compassionate and encouraging words to myself today.
"For as he thinketh in his heart, so is he" (Prov. 23:7).
(For as she thinks in her heart, so is she.)

Words have power.
"Death and life are in the power of the tongue" (Prov. 18:23).

Acknowledge your feelings, and then speak what you want.
This is very challenging for me, but I will be okay. I will learn how to live with fluctuating hormones.

Even though I don't feel like it, I have the ability to be patient with others today.

I am feeling alone in this, but I know millions of women are going through this too.

I am feeling depressed, but these feelings are temporary and will pass.

My neighbor doesn't struggle like I do, but I will not compare myself to her.

I am tired, but I will make it through this day.

44

I do not like these emotional days, but I will think about what is good in my life.

I am feeling so out of control! I will keep today simple, do what I can, and know that whatever I don't get done, it will be okay, somehow!

I am not sure what to do, but I will give today to God and ask Him for wisdom.

I feel like a loser today, but despite how I feel, I am who God says I am; as righteous as Jesus Christ.

Karen Turner

RECOMMENDED READING

BOOKS
The Bible

The Wisdom of Menopause by Christiane Northrup, MD

Embracing Menopause Naturally by Gabriele Kushi

The Silent Passage by Gail Sheehy

The Slow Down Diet by Marc David

Female Brain Gone Insane: An Emergency Guide For Women Who Feel Like They Are Falling Apart by Mia Lundin, R.N.C., and N.P.

The Mood Cure and The Diet Cure by Julia Ross, MA

The 4:8 Principle by Tommy Newberry

WEBSITE ARTICLES
http://www.johnleemd.com/physiological-effects-estrogen-progesterone.html

http://www.truthortradition.com/articles/suffering-well

www.AndreaBeaman.com

https://www.hormonesbalance.com/quiz/

http://www.chrisheinz.com/read/post/7_benefits_of_praising_god

https://www.cru.org/train-and-grow/spiritual-growth/devotionals/why-every-christian-should-keep-a-journal.html

http://psychcentral.com/lib/the-health-benefits-of-journaling/

AUTHOR BIOGRAPHY

Karen Turner is a certified holistic health coach, licensed massage therapist, member of the American Association of Drugless Practitioners, and author. She received her nutrition training from the Institute for Integrative Nutrition and American Health Science University. Karen works with people who would like to improve their health but are feeling stuck due to the confusing information about food and dieting. Clients describe her as "empathetic, insightful, and motivating." For information about health coaching and recipes, visit www.KarenLTurner.com.

This book was inspired by my experience at the Institute for Integrative Nutrition® (IIN) where I received my training in holistic wellness and health coaching. IIN offers a truly comprehensive Health Coach Training Program that invites students to deeply explore the things that are most nourishing to them. From the physical aspects of nutrition and eating wholesome foods that work best for each individual person, to the concept of Primary Food – the idea that everything in life including our spirituality, career, relationships, and fitness contribute to our inner and outer health - IIN helped me reach optimal health and balance. This inner journey unleashed the passion that compelled me to share what I've learned and inspire others.

Beyond personal health, IIN offers training in health coaching, as well as business and marketing training. Students, who choose to pursue this field professionally, complete the program equipped with the communication skills and branding knowledge they need to create a fulfilling career encouraging and supporting others reach their own health goals.

From renowned wellness experts as Visiting Teachers to the convenience of their online learning platform, this school has changed my life and I believe it will do the same for you. I invite you to learn more about the Institute for Integrative Nutrition and explore how the Health Coach Training Program can help you transform your life. Feel free to contact me to hear more about my personal experience at www.KarenLTurner.com or call (844) 315-8546 to learn more.

www.ingramcontent.com/pod-product-compliance
Lightning Source LLC
Chambersburg PA
CBHW070128290526

45789CB00005B/2158